Natália M. Bustamante Sá
Paula M. Guttmann

Traumatic Septic Arthritis in an Equine Tarsus

Natália M. Bustamante Sá
Paula M. Guttmann

Traumatic Septic Arthritis in an Equine Tarsus

Case Report

ScienciaScripts

Imprint
Any brand names and product names mentioned in this book are subject to trademark, brand or patent protection and are trademarks or registered trademarks of their respective holders. The use of brand names, product names, common names, trade names, product descriptions etc. even without a particular marking in this work is in no way to be construed to mean that such names may be regarded as unrestricted in respect of trademark and brand protection legislation and could thus be used by anyone.

Cover image: www.ingimage.com

This book is a translation from the original published under ISBN 978-613-9-60213-1.

Publisher:
Sciencia Scripts
is a trademark of
Dodo Books Indian Ocean Ltd. and OmniScriptum S.R.L publishing group

120 High Road, East Finchley, London, N2 9ED, United Kingdom
Str. Armeneasca 28/1, office 1, Chisinau MD-2012, Republic of Moldova, Europe
Printed at: see last page
ISBN: 978-620-7-26983-9

"Some horses will test you, some will teach you, and some will bring out the best in you." Author: Unknown

ACKNOWLEDGEMENTS

I would like to thank all those who contributed to this work, especially my mother Eloisa Elena Murga Martins and my father Paulo César Bustamante Sá (*In memoriam*), Maria Eduarda Monteiro Silva and Paula de Mattos Guttmann for their patience, encouragement and teachings.

Index

CHAPTER 1

INTRODUCTION

The locomotor system is responsible for the support, locomotion, structure and stability of animals. In horses, this is the basis for the leverage system exerted by the joints. Of the 205 bones that make up the horse, 40 are present in the back of the animal, which is the region that provides the most impetus, so the joints that are usually affected by injuries are the intertarsal and tarsometatarsal joints.The horse's well-being is directly proportional to the health of its locomotor system, which needs to be intact and functional. However, this will be affected if there are any disturbances in this system, such as lameness and chronic pain, thus impairing its performance, generating loss of function or even creating situations incompatible with the life of an animal that reaches around 500kg by the time it reaches adulthood.These osteoarticular alterations, such as septic arthritis, can negatively affect a foal's future if the necessary intervention measures are not taken, since the paediatric phase is among the most critical, especially when the affected area is the musculoskeletal system.Traumas are among the most frequent occurrences in foals and young horses, most of which live on pasture. Veterinary care needs to be provided immediately, regardless of the severity of the injury, to ensure that the patient's clinical condition does not worsen and consequently reduce the chances of drastic and chronic consequences occurring, thus ensuring greater longevity for the animal.

In view of the above, this paper aims to report the case of a foal affected by septic arthritis as a result of trauma.

CHAPTER 2

LITERATURE REVIEW

2.1 MORPHOFUNCTIONAL ASPECTS OF THE TARSAL JOINT

2.1.1 Anatomy

The equine tarsus, commonly known as the "hock", is made up of the talus, the calcaneus, the central tarsal bone, the first and second tarsal bones, which are fused, and the third and fourth tarsal bones (KAINER, 2006), with the calcaneus being the largest structure present (PALMEIRA, 2008). The talus, which is also called the astragalus or tarsal-tibial bone, has a continuous proximal surface, forming the trochlea which articulates with the distal end of the tibia. The calcaneus, or tarsofibular bone, is characterised by being elongated and transversely flattened. Its distal end has a concave face that articulates with the fourth tarsal bone (GETTY, 1986; COSTA 2012).

The central tarsal bone is located between the talus, where it articulates proximally, and the third tarsal, where it articulates distally. The first and second tarsal bones are located on the medioplantar surface, distal to the central bone. The fourth tarsal bone is arranged laterally in the distal layer, where the proximal surface articulates with the calcaneus, the distal surface with the third and fourth metatarsals and the medial surface articulates with the central bone and the third tarsal bone (Figure 01) (GETTY, 1986).

However, these bones on their own don't allow for as much movement as the knee, for example. It is therefore the strong ligaments present in this region that will facilitate movement (SELLNOW, 2017).The ligaments have the function of maintaining the stability of the joint, distributing the forces exerted equally, and are made up of collagen fibres. The collateral ligaments are associated with the joint capsule and the intra-articular ligaments normally cover the synovial membrane (MCILWRAITH, 2001).

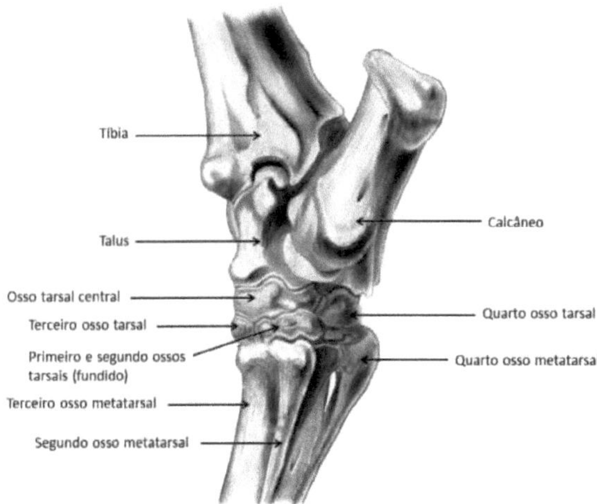

Figure 01 - Caudomedial view of the equine tarsus
Source: Adapted from Inkymousestudios.com, 2015.

The long lateral collateral ligament extends from the lateral malleolus of the tibia and attaches distally to the calcaneus, the fourth tarsal bone, the talus and the third and fourth metatarsal bones. Fused to this ligament is the tendon of the lateral digital extensor muscle. The three short lateral collateral ligaments insert into the lateral malleolus (TARTANIUK, 2017).

The long medial collateral ligament of the tarsus has a proximal insertion in the medial tibial malleolus, extending distally and dividing into a superficial layer that passes through the cunean tendon (medial tendon) and inserts into the fused bones of the tarsus and the proximal ends of the second and third metatarsal bones, and a deep layer that attaches distally to the distal tuberosity of the talus and the central and third tarsal bones. The superficial short medial collateral ligament runs from the medial tibial malleolus to the tuberosities of the talus and central tarsal bone (KAINER, 2006; TARTANIUK, 2017).

The dorsal tarsal ligament originates from the distal tuberosity of the talus and inserts into the central tarsal bone, the third tarsal bone and the proximal region of the third metatarsal.

The long plantar tarsal ligament is also present, coming from the calcaneus and inserting into the fourth metatarsal and the fourth tarsal bone (TARTANIUK, 2017).

These ligaments will fuse with the fibrous capsule of the tarsal joints, which is thinner dorsally and thicker on the plantar and distal sides. The cartilage of the capsule will provide a softer surface for the deep digital flexor tendon, preventing friction and enabling it to perform to its full potential. The gastrocnemius tendon inserts into the plantar part of the calcaneal tuberosity, while the tendons of the superficial digital flexor, biceps femoris and semitendinosus muscles insert dorsally into the same structure (Figure 02) (KAINER, 2006).

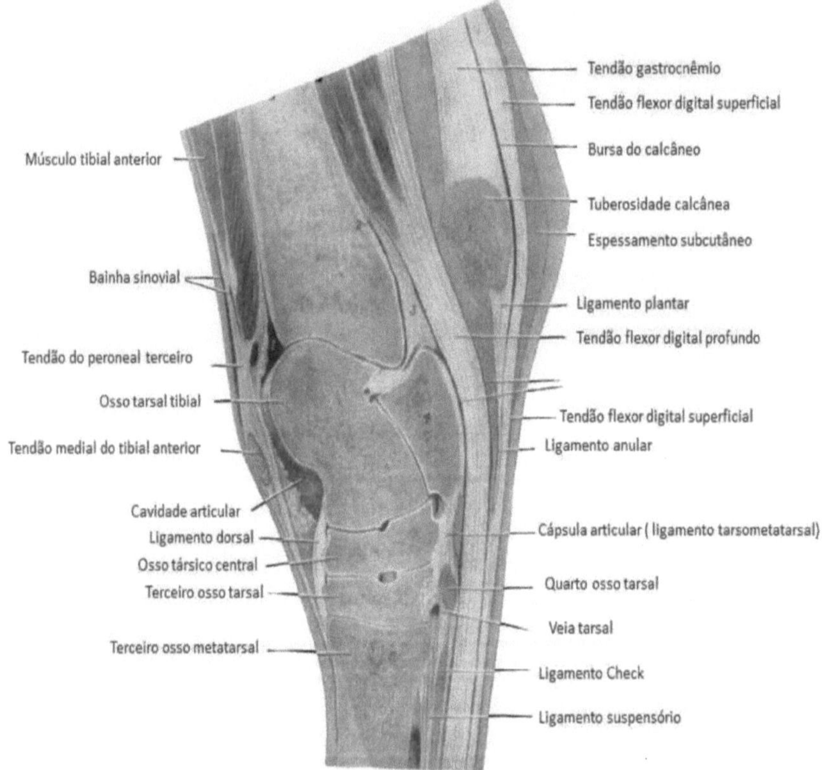

Figure 02 - Longitudinal section of the tarsal region of an equine, illustrating the ligaments and tendons
Source: Adapted from Kate, 2012.

The equine tarsus is made up of four joints: tibiotarsal, proximal intertarsal, distal intertarsal and tarsometatarsal (Figure 03) (ALVES, 2008).

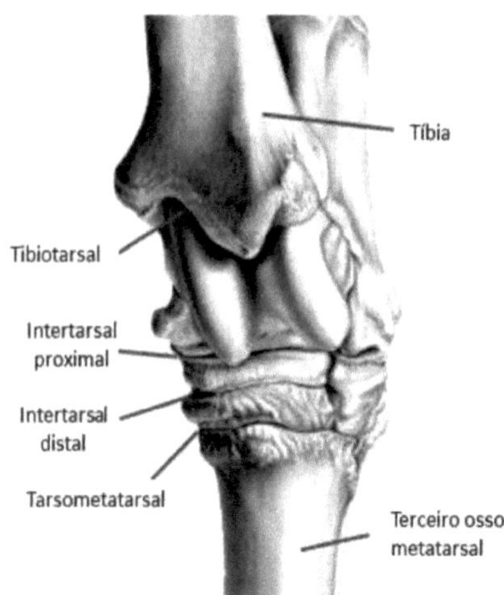

Figure 03 - Craniolateral view of the tarsal joints
Source: Adapted from Atlantaequine.com, 2016.

The trochlea of the talus articulates proximally with the cochlear surface of the tibia, resulting in the formation of the tibiotarsal joint (KAINER, 2006), which normally has a synovial fossa characterised by a well-defined depression in the central portion of the intertrochlear cleft of the talus bone, which is absent in young foals (GALLO, 2010). It is also the joint with the greatest flexion power (JACKMAN, 2006), since the other three practically don't move (MILLER, 2017). The tibiotarsal joint is flexed by contraction of the cranial tibial muscle and traction of the third peroneal tendon muscle, where the gastrocnemius, biceps femoris and semitendinosus muscles are also present in the extension of this joint (KAINER, 2006).

The proximal intertarsal joint communicates with the tibiotarsal joint (DYCE; SACK; WENSING, 2010), but has no communication with the distal intertarsal joint (ALVES, 2008). The distal intertarsal joint is proximally bordered by the central tarsal bone and distally by the third, first and second tarsal bones. Extending laterally to this joint is the fourth tarsal bone, which articulates with the proximal intertarsal and tarsometatarsal joints, situated between the distal layer of the tarsal bones and proximal to the metatarsal bone (JACKMAN, 2006).

2.1.2 Joint structure

According to Todhunter (1996) the joint is made up of bone, articular cartilage, fibrous joint capsule, synovial membrane and synovial fluid (Figure 04).

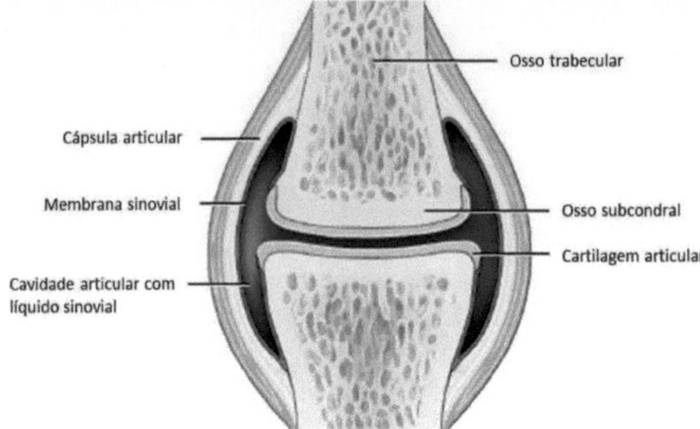

Figure 04 - Schematic representation of a joint
Source: Adapted from Weeren, 2016.

2.1.2.a Subchondral bone

Subchondral bone provides support, stability and prevention of damage to articular cartilage, and can undergo remodelling according to the amount of weight deposited under the joint. Its constitution includes inorganic compounds such as hydroxyapatite crystals ($Ca10(PO4)6(OH)2$), which guarantee hardness and resistance. Organic compounds such as proteoglycans, type I collagen, glycosaminoglycans and water provide flexibility and resistance to subchondral bone (KAWCAK, 2016).

Other important compounds are cytokines, TNF-α (tumour necrosis factor α, interleukins and IFN- γ (interferon γ). When the subcondral bone is affected by a disease, these cytokines are released and the articular cartilage is exposed to them, which can lead to lesions that compromise the joint (TODHUNTER, 1996; MCILWRAITH, 2006).

2.1.2.b Articular cartilage

Articular cartilage has an opaque, milky appearance in the thicker regions and a translucent appearance in the thinner regions, due to the high concentration of water in its constitution (70% - 80%). Other compounds are proteoglycans (PGs), collagens, glycoproteins, minerals and lipids which are present in the four layers of cartilage: the tangential or superficial layer, the intermediate or transition layer, the radiated or deep layer and the calcified layer. The tangential layer has flattened chondrocytes, densely arranged type II collagen fibres and a low amount of PGs with a high concentration of water; the intermediate layer contains a low amount of water, a higher concentration of PGs and less dense collagens; the radiated layer has more rounded chondrocytes dispersed irregularly in the extracellular matrix and the calcified layer is characterised by having less collagen, a high concentration of PGs, less water and chondrocytes arranged in columns perpendicular to the subchondral bone (WEEREN, 2016).

In horses, the articular cartilage is generally hyaline, which allows mobility and weight bearing without friction, but fibrocartilage can be found at the junction of the articular cartilage, in the synovial membrane, in the periosteum and in the meniscus (MCILWRAITH, 2006; RIJT, 2011).

During the animal's development, cartilage growth slows down as the ossification process progresses, leading to an advance of the ossification zone towards the articular cartilage, resulting in a thinner aspect of the chondrocyte germ layer (GALLO, 2010).

Collagens act in the structure of articular cartilage by forming fibres and fibrils interwoven throughout the matrix, and are responsible for providing the elastic strength required by the cartilage. The arrangement of their architecture can change depending on the zone in question or the depth at which they are found in the cartilage. Around sixteen types of collagen have been described in mammalian species and can be divided into two main categories: collagen-forming fibrils (types I, II, III, V and XI) and non-collagen-forming fibrils (FRISBIE, 2012).

In horses, the elastic force is exerted by the superficial layer, where the fibres are oriented parallel to the joint surface. It has been shown that collagen synthesis occurs more significantly in adult animals when compared to younger ones (RIJT, 2011).

Still with regard to the constitution of articular cartilage, proteoglycans are the most fundamental substances in cartilage and are characterised by being a chondromucoid gel made up of proteins, glycosaminoglycans, hyaluronic acid, chondroitin A and B, lactates, mineral salts, calcium and water. Proteoglycans are hydrophilic, i.e. they bind to water molecules and thus play an important role in the transport of water and electrolytes. They can also bind to tropocollagen molecules and take part in the production of collagen fibres (ALVES, 2008).

The importance of proteoglycans lies not only in their properties, but also in their function of giving articular cartilage physical and chemical resistance and the ability to permeate (SOUZA; PINHAL, 2017).

The glycoproteins that also play a role in cartilage formation are binding proteins such as chondronectin, which participates in the adhesion of chondrocytes to the surface of type II collagen, fibronectin, adhesion of cells to molecules and surfaces and the oligomeric cartilage matrix protein (VENDRUSCOLO, 2011).

Chondrocytes, on the other hand, make up a small portion of the cartilage, but they have an important function, which is to maintain the synthesis of the extracellular matrix. These have been shown to be extremely sensitive to changes in the extracellular composition of the matrix, changes that result from catabolism and/or physical stimuli as well as the ageing of the animal, with the production of proteolytic enzymes that have a degradative effect on the matrix (TODHUNTER, 1996).

2.1.2.c Fibrous articular capsule

The joint capsule consists of a fibrous portion that aligns with the lamina propria and synovial membrane, maintaining contact with the synovial fluid. This portion is made up of a dense fibrous tissue that ensures the mechanical stability of the joint by inserting itself into the adjacent bone (MCILWRAITH, 2001). This fibrous portion has a wide variety of nerve endings, through which joint pain is detected (VIEIRA, 2009).

2.1.2.d Synovial membrane

The cells of the synovial membrane are the major sources of synovial fluid components, acting as a semi-permeable membrane and responsible for controlling molecules entering and/or leaving the joint space, thus playing an essential role in preserving the physiology of articular cartilage (NEUENSCHWANDER, 2016).

Under normal conditions, high molecular weight molecules such as hyaluronic acid and lubricin are not rapidly permeable, while small molecules such as growth factors and cytokines are rapidly diffused through the synovial membrane. This prevents large molecules from depositing on the joint surface and causing changes in the viscosity and composition of the synovial fluid (SCANZELLO; GOLDRING, 2012).

This is a flexible membrane that ensures joint movement (DURHAM; DYSON, 2003) by interacting directly with the synovial fluid (MOLLER; WEEREN, 2017), acting to facilitate its diffusion (THOMSEN et al., 2017) and covering the entire joint surface, except for the articular cartilage and some areas of the bones. The synovial membrane is a non-uniform vascular tissue and denser tissue can be found in areas prone to trauma (CARON, 2003).

The cellular elements that make up the synovial membrane act as a source for the compounds in the synovial fluid, contributing to the unique properties of the joint surface and modulating the activity of the chondrocytes (SCANZELLO; GOLDRING, 2012). It consists of two layers: the intima and the subintima. The first layer ensures an incomplete cellular lining and is located close to the joint cavity, overlying a deeper layer of connective tissue called the subintima. This second layer consists of loose connective tissue containing numerous blood vessels (MCILWRAITH, 2006).

The intimal layer is made up of synovial cells, which are called synoviocytes and are classified according to their ultrastructure into three types: A, B and C, where type A resembles macrophages and plays a phagocytic role; type B resembles fibroblasts and is the most abundant, synthesising a wide variety of macromolecules, including collagen; and type C is intermediate between the other two (CARON, 2003).

As a result of an inflammatory response by the synovial membrane, there will be a drop in the synthesis of chondrocytes and the release of catabolic mediators resulting in the breakdown of homeostasis and degradation of articular cartilage

(GRAUW et al., 2011).

2.1.2. and Synovial Fluid

The components of the synovial fluid or synovial liquid are derived from the plasma ultrafiltrate, which comes from the capillaries present in the synovial membrane (TODHUNTER, 1996), contributing to the functionality of the articular surface and modulating the activity of the chondrocytes (NEUENSCHWANDER, 2016) and participating in the transport of nutrients that reach the articular cartilage (FONSECA et al., 2009).

It has a light yellow or colourless colour, mononucleated and polymorphonucleated cells and high viscosity due to the presence of hyaluronic acid, which is the main component of synovial fluid and is responsible for sliding the synovial membrane over the opposing surface. In horses, changes in these characteristics can suggest a joint disorder, indicating the relative amount of synovitis, following a range of inflammatory activity in the joint (MCILWRAITH, 2006).

The lubricating property comes from a mucin-like glycoprotein called lubricin, also known as proteoglycan 4, which is secreted by chondrocytes, synoviocytes and cells in the meniscus. This glycoprotein adheres to the surface of the articular cartilage and to the synovial membrane, reducing tension on the articular surface (SVALA et al., 2015).

2.2 SEPTIC ARTHRITIS
2.2.1 **Definition**

The term septic arthritis refers to the presence of microorganisms in the synovial space of a joint, generating a process of severe inflammation. This condition can result in the destruction of articular cartilage and joint dysfunction. It can occur by haematogenous, iatrogenic or traumatic means (MEIJER; WEEREN; RIJKENHUIZEN, 2000).

Haematogenous infection in foals is the biggest cause of morbidity and mortality. Its occurrence can be related to a failure in the passive transfer of antibodies, respiratory tract disorders, umbilical diseases or gastrointestinal infections. These problems can ensure that the microorganism is inoculated into the synovial membrane of a joint via the bloodstream, which can lead to septicaemia (GLASS; WATTS, 2017).

The iatrogenic route can be through joint puncture procedures or the administration of intra-articular medication (HUNTER; BLYTH, 1999). Intra-articular medication can lead to septic arthritis and an acute aseptic inflammatory process, described as pseudo-septic arthritis, although this is uncommon (STEEL; PANNIRSELVAM; ANDERSON, 2013).

Traumatic injuries, on the other hand, occur when bacteria enter the joint space as a result of perforative or penetrative trauma (SHIRTLIFF; MADER, 2002). This trauma is usually related to lacerations, and the most commonly affected joint is the tibiotarsal joint. The infectious agent gains access to the joint capsule, reaching the synovial fluid (CARTER, 1991).

2.2.2 Etiopathogenesis

Preferably, joints and their adjacent tissues are the ideal places for microorganisms to settle and proliferate, especially in foals under six months of age. This is due to the low blood flow and low oxygen tension in the tissues around the joint (MORTON, 2005). Once a trauma has occurred, the pathogen enters the joint space generating a severe process of inflammation, resulting in the production of inflammatory mediators that are largely responsible for the clinical signs and damage caused to the joint (SUTTER; BERTONE, 2007), as well as an increase and infiltration of polymorphonucleated cells, such as neutrophils; the release of cytokines that act on chondrocytes and synoviocytes and proteolytic enzymes that contribute to vascular congestion, preventing vascularisation of the subchondral bone and generating alterations in the dynamics of the synovial fluid and its effusion. All these mechanisms contribute to the destruction of articular cartilage, through proteolytic enzymes and malnutrition of this cartilage, since the production of synovial fluid will be impaired (ANNEAR; FURR; WHITE, 2011).

Over the course of the infection, the longer it lasts, the greater the likelihood of permanent damage to the synovial structure and degradation of the articular cartilage, due to the presence of lysosomal enzymes, neutrophils, metalloproteinases, collagenases and hyaluronidases (SCHNEIDER, 1998). Damage to the synovial fluid can occur early on, even before clinical signs are present, and can prevent the synovial membrane from performing its function correctly, directly interfering with the nutrition of the chondrocytes.

In addition, there is a risk of developing abnormalities in the articular cartilage, resulting in the loss of proteoglycans and exposing this cartilage to deteriorating mechanisms and the action of degradation enzymes. Once destroyed, the damage to the cartilage is irreversible, characterising the final stage of septic arthritis, contributing to the impediment of the joint's anatomical function (BAXTER, 2008).

As Motta et al. (2017) state, many animals quickly develop a chronic condition, resulting in loss of joint movement and a tendency to remain in a recumbent position.

When microorganisms are present in the joint, the lesions caused by these pathogens are highly pyogenic, hinder tissue repair and usually do not respond significantly to treatment with conventional antibiotics, evolving into chronic septic arthritis (QUINN et al., 2011).

The synovial membrane will respond to this inflammatory and infectious condition through hyperaemia resulting from increased vascular permeability, causing fibrin to leak out along with macrophage efflux. During the course of the infection, there can also be an increase in the production of interleukins (IL-1β and IL-6) as well as TNF-α and the presence of joint effusion with a significant increase in the sensitivity of the joint capsule (WEEREN, 2016), which because it contains many nociceptors that extend to the synovial membrane generates a lot of pain, which can be intensified by the release of prostaglandin E2 from the inflammatory cascade (ANNEAR; FURR; WHITE, 2011). In addition, there is a reduction in blood flow in the joint capsule, generating ischaemia in the adjacent tissues and contributing to an excessive production of fibrin, which if not removed persists in the joint for several weeks. The accumulation of this fibrin promotes the formation of a fibrinocellular conglomerate in the intrasynovial space which acts to cover and trap bacteria, foreign bodies and/or devitalised tissues, contributing to the continuation of inflammation and the destructive effects of its cycle (MORTON, 2005).

The types of lesions in foals can be described according to their location in the joint or in the bone, so they can be classified as: synovial lesions (Type S), located in a joint with involvement of the synovial structures without reaching the bone; lesions in the epiphyses (Type E), occurring in the subchondral bone adjacent to the articular cartilage; infection in the physis (Type P), involving the metaphysis of the affected bone (PARADIS, 2006) and lesion of the tarsal bones (Type T), seen in premature foals (HARDY, 2006).

A number of pathogens are associated with septic arthritis, with bacteria being the most prevalent. Foals are the most susceptible to bacterial infections, most of which are caused by: *Escherichia coli*, *Actinobacillus*, *Klebsiella spp*, *Rhodococcus equi*, *Streptococcus spp and Staphylococcus spp* (WARREN et al., 2015). These pathogens can be transmitted after trauma, through direct contact by breaking the skin or mucous membranes, as well as indirect contact through contaminated environments (HIBER; DARLING, 2012). With regard to *Staphylococcus spp,* it has been experimentally proven that 1.5×10^5 and 1.6×10^6 colony forming units (CFU) are capable of causing infection in the tibiotarsal joint of healthy horses (BAXTER, 2008). In addition to these pathogens, *Salmonella spp.* may also be present as a causative agent of septic arthritis (GLASS; WATTS, 2017).

The involvement of bacteria in the infectious and inflammatory process is directly related to extracellular virulence (ABDELNOUR et al., 1993), components of the bacterial cell wall, such as the existence of protein A in *Staphylococcus spp* (PALMQVIST et al., 2005), peptides mediating neutrophil recruitment that contribute to joint damage (GJERTSSON et al., 2012) or even oligonucleotide sequences present in bacterial DNA (DENG; TARKOWSKI, 2000).

2.2.3 Epidemiology

Puncture trauma to the synovial cavity is a well-reported complicating factor in horses, and joints close to the trauma are usually affected by septic arthritis (SCHNEIDER et al., 1992).

According to Weeren (2016), the tibiotarsal joint is the most affected (34 per cent), followed by the metacarpophalangeal/metatarsophalangeal (20 per cent), carpal (18 per cent) and patellofemoral (9 per cent) joints.

Although septic arthritis affects all large animals, it is better known in horses due to the great importance of the locomotor system in this species, and is considered one of the most serious joint problems. In foals, the greatest risk of infection is during the first month of life, which may be due to a partial or complete failure in the passive transfer of immunoglobulins, especially in neonatal foals and may not be related to septicaemia (RIZZONI; MIYAUCHI, 2012; WEEREN, 2016).

Infection will depend on a number of factors, such as the size of the inoculum, the host's defence, the virulence of the microorganism and which joint has been affected (HARDY, 2006). All these factors can increase the risk of morbidity and mortality in foals (VOS; DUCHARME, 2008), where the reported rates are 5.2% and 27.4%, respectively (EASLEY et al., 2011), which may be due to difficulties in the recovery process from already established infections and/or because there is degenerative damage associated with the inflammation process (LUDWIG et al., 2016).

The incidence of septic arthritis after arthroscopy is 0.9%. This figure is confirmed in cases where there was no prophylaxis during the surgical procedure, and is directly related to the animal's period of hospitalisation (BORG; CARMALT, 2013).

Medicines administered intra-articularly can become risk factors, contributing to the development of septic arthritis. This is due to the wrong method of treatment and choice of drug, and it has been proven that the use of corticosteroids such as betamethasone has a risk of developing septic arthritis.
lower when compared to the use of dexamethasone. One in every 1249 cases of septic arthritis is due to the improper administration of medication in a joint (STEEL; PANNIRSELVAM; ANDERSON, 2013).

2.2.4 **Symptomatology**

Animals affected by septic arthritis usually show lameness, high fever, apathy, prostration, periarticular oedema (Figure 05), joint pain, local changes such as distension and changes in the colour of the skin around the joint involved, fistulas and secondary wounds (RIZZONI, MIYAUCHI, 2012). They may also present joint effusion, cellulitis and increased intra-articular fluid, which may not be detected due to the small size of the joint capsule, very characteristic of tarsal joints (SCHNEIDER, 2006). Foals can also show moderate to severe laminitis, which varies according to the size of the animal, but is not always present (VOS; DUCHARME, 2008).

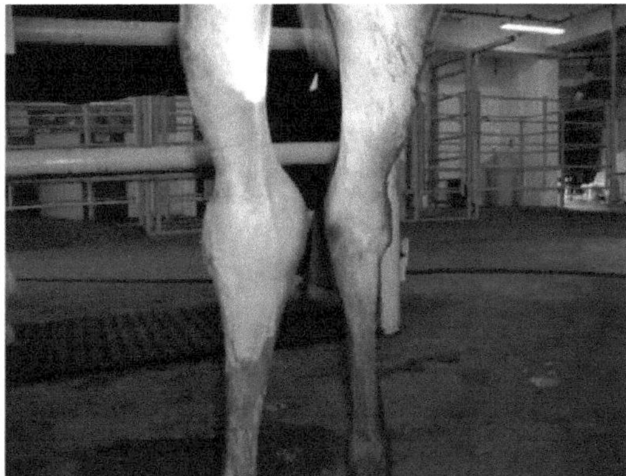

Figure 05 - Oedema in the tarsal region of the right hind limb in a foal
Source: Vieira, 2009.

2.2.5 **Diagnosis**

Analysis of synovial fluid is extremely important in cases of septic arthritis, which in many cases has a characteristic bloody colour, slightly cloudy to opaque and with reduced viscosity (Figure 06) (GLASS; WATTS, 2017). Dark yellow or light amber samples (xanthochromic) represent previous haemorrhage and may be associated with chronic traumatic arthritis. If the liquid collected is opaque and contains flocculent material, it indicates synovitis, which may be related to infectious arthritis, resulting in a serofibrinous to fibropurulent sample (VIEIRA, 2009).

According to Barber (2008), when a joint is inflamed and/or contains microorganisms, the synovial fluid will contain a high number of white cells ($> 30 \times 10^9$

/ L), neutrophils (> 80%) and a high concentration of proteins (> 4.0g/dL).

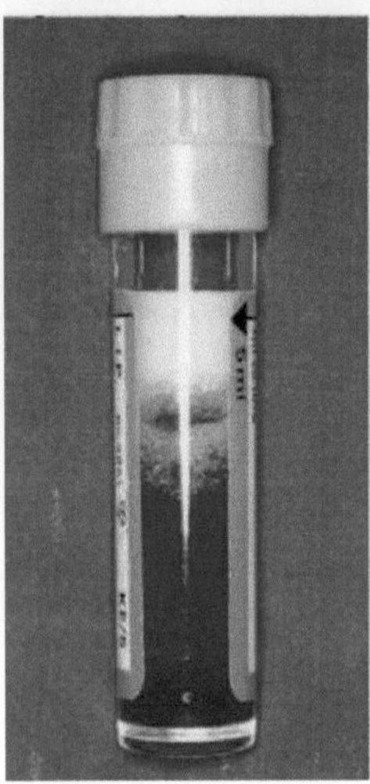

Figure 06 - Synovial fluid obtained from a septic joint with a bloody appearance
Source: Weeren, 2017.

This fluid can be obtained by aspiration via arthrocentesis (Figure 07). Sometimes several attempts are necessary due to the angle of needle insertion and palpation of the right site (BODAAN; RILEY; ENGELI, 2017). This is an aseptic procedure in which the collected fluid is placed in a tube containing ethylenediamine tetraacetic acid (EDTA) for cytology and antimicrobial culture (ANNEAR; FURR; WHITE, 2011).

An important factor to be analysed in synovial fluid is serum amyloid A (SAA), as it is a marker for septic arthritis. This protein does not change in concentration during arthrocentesis, intra-articular administration of amikacin or during arthroscopy. Normally, its level is undetectable or very low in healthy animals, but during the course of the disease its concentration in the synovial fluid is high (100-150 mg/L) (JACOBSEN; THOMSEN; NANNI, 2006).

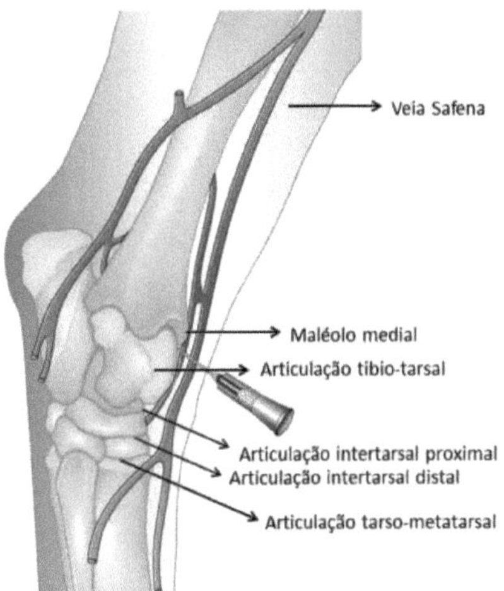

Figure 07 - Arthrocentesis of the tibio-tarsal joint in a horse
Source: Adapted from Rodgerson, 2008.

Radiography is a very important diagnostic method, especially in foals, as there is an increased likelihood that bones adjacent to the affected joint will be affected. In the first few days of infection, the image will not reveal much or any data, as the joint and bones are usually normal (Figure 08). However, during the course of the infection and as the acute phase progresses to the chronic phase, the following findings may be seen: increased volume of the joint capsule and soft tissues around the joint, displacement of fatty tissue, increased joint space due to oedema and effusion (SHIRTLIFF; MADER, 2002). Signs such as the accumulation of air inside the joint, fractures associated with the onset of sepsis, periosteal proliferation, thickening of the subcutaneous and capsular tissues, foreign bodies, osteomyelitis, sequestration or alterations to the joint surface, bone lysis, periarticular oedema, distension of the joint capsule and marginal osteolysis may be present (Figure 09) (VIEIRA, 2009). In addition, loss of joint space due to loss of cartilage, lysis of subchondral bone and the presence of osteophytes are very common findings in septic arthritis, especially in the chronic stage (MOSTAFA; ABU-SEIDA; EL-GLIL, 2014).

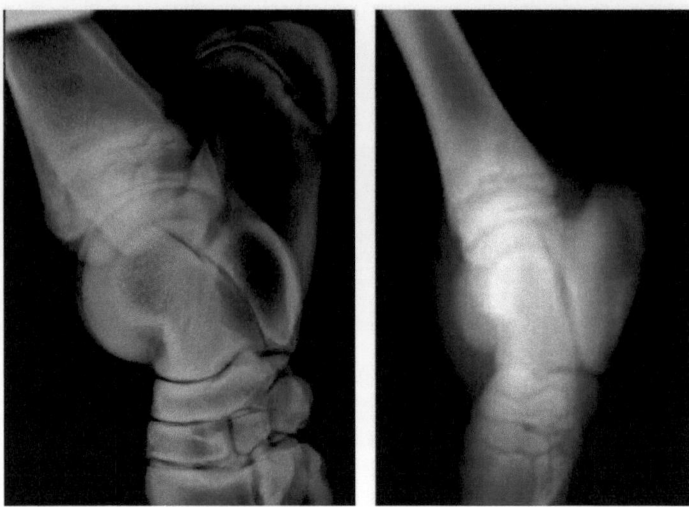
Figure 08 - Equine tarsal region without anomaly
Figure 09 - Oblique view of an equine tarsus showing bone lysis, an area of sclerosis in the distal part of the tibia and joint distension
Source: Adapted from Cavecreekequine.com, Source: Adapted from Sayegh, 2001. 2016.

Imaging diagnostic techniques are very important in assessing joint infection. As well as radiography, ultrasound can also be used to assess periarticular wounds, check for joint effusion, synovial fluid characteristics such as the existence of an inflammatory process, the presence of foreign bodies and whether there is soft tissue involvement. The findings can be: thickening of the synovial membrane, effusion with hyperechogenic particles, cellularity (echogenic or hypoechogenic) and fibrin deposition resulting in an image with echogenic material (Figure 10 and 11) (BECCATI et.al., 2015).

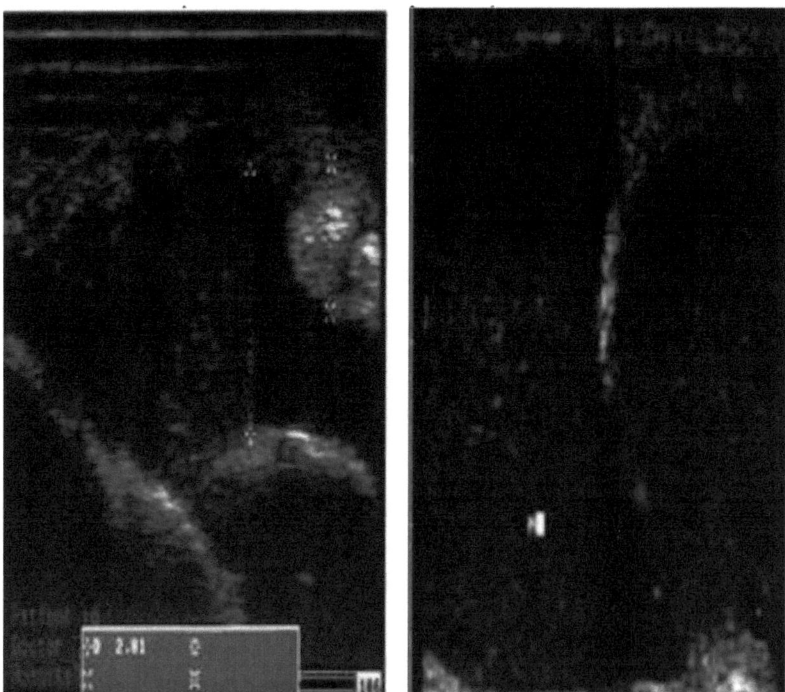

Figure 10 - Dorsomedial view of the tibiotarsal joint containing anechoic fluid and a hypoechoic mass
Figure 11 - Medial view of the tibiotarsal joint containing anechoic fluid and synovial proliferation
Source: Mostafa; Abu-seida; El-glil, 2014. Source: Mostafa; Abu-seida; El-glil, 2014.

In foals with septic arthritis, it is common to see bone lesions as hyperintense images with a hypointense halo (Figure 12). Interpretation of the results varies according to the intensity of the signal emitted during the examination, which includes the metaphysis, physis, epiphysis, articular cartilage and synovial fluid, regardless of the foal's age and anatomical region (GASCHEN et al., 2011).

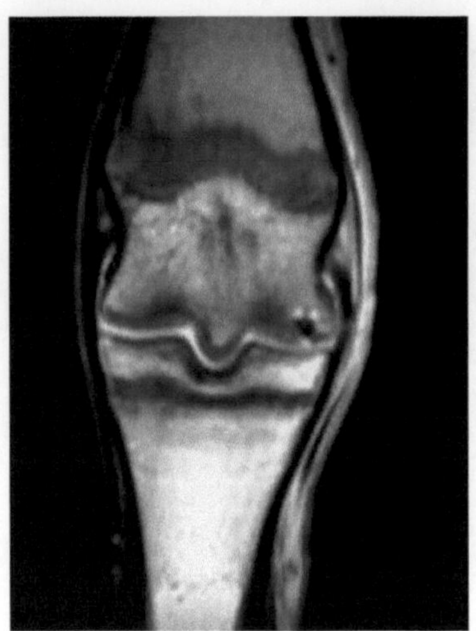

Figure 12 - MRI scan, dorsal view of the metatarsal, showing a lesion on the lateral condyle of the third metatarsal and a subchondral lesion
Source: Gaschen et al., 2011.

Computed tomography is a resource that can be used to help diagnose septic arthritis, visualising soft tissues and bones, including distal aspects of the middle phalanx, distal phalanx and navicular bone (PORTER; WERPY, 2014). However, it is not widely used in cases of joint infection, even though it offers some advantages over radiography, with greater sensitivity and a wealth of detail, being efficient in detecting the initial signs of septic arthritis, such as thickening of the synovial membrane and possible joint effusions (ANNEAR; FURR; WHITE, 2011).

Another technique is arthroscopy, which allows the visualisation of fibrin debris, synovial necrosis, detached cartilage fragments, regions of adhesions, fissures, joint degeneration, hypertrophy of the synovial villi and erosion with irregularity of the joint surface (Figures 13, 14, 15 and 16) (MOSTAFA; ABU- SEIDA; EL-GLIL, 2014).

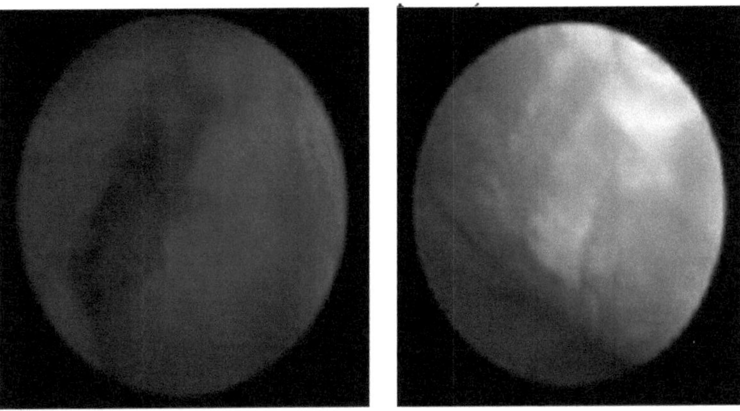

Figure 13 - Digital arthroscopy of the tibiotarsal joint with erosion of the articular surface
Figure 14 - Digital arthroscopy of the tibiotarsal joint showing   the presence of a fissure
Source: Adapted from Mostafa; Abu-seida; El-glil, 2014.

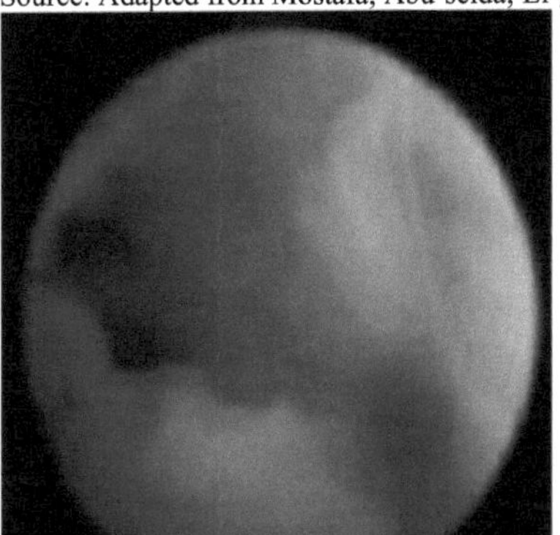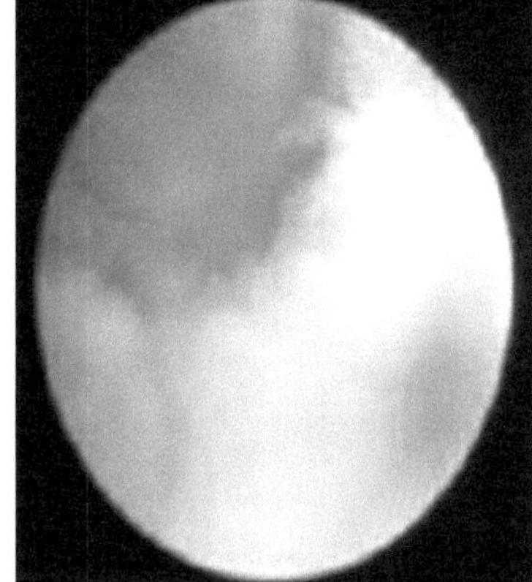

Figure 15 - Digital arthroscopy of the tibiotarsal joint showing joint degeneration
Figure 16 - Digital arthroscopy of the tibiotarsal joint with hypertrophy of the synovial villi
Source: Adapted from Mostafa; Abu- seida; El-glil, 2014.

2.2.6 **Treatment**

Among the existing forms of treatment for septic arthritis is arthroscopy. This is used to remove fibrin, debris, treat proliferative synovitis, intra-articular fractures and ruptures and avulsions of the joint capsule, especially in the tibiotarsal joint (Figure 17) (MCILWRAITH; NIXON; WRIGHT, 2015).

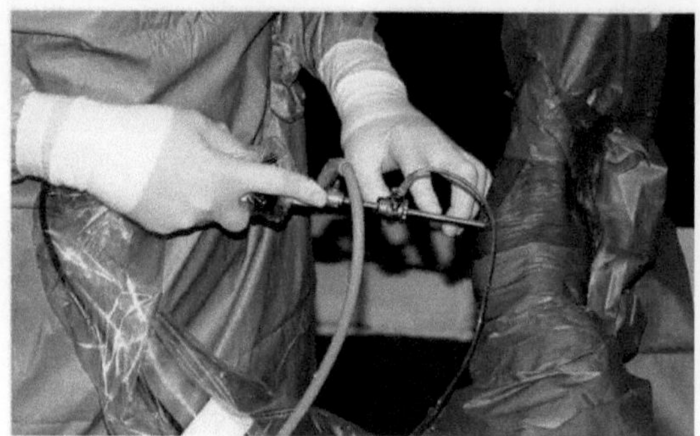
Figure 17 - Dorsomedial arthroscopy of the tibiotarsal joint in a horse
Source: Mcilwraith et al., 2015.

It is generally a low-risk procedure (BORG; CARMALT, 2013) that uses gas or a liquid medium to distend the joint. Normally, the fluids used are balanced-polyionic hydrogen potential (pH) solutions, such as ringer's lactate (FISCHER et al., 2006).

This is a technique that ensures small incisions in the joint, allowing better exploration of the area, removing products produced by bacteria that may be in the synovial tissue of the joint capsule, reducing post-operative time and minimising problems such as suture dehiscence (CABLE, 2017).

Arthroscopy is widely used in cases of chronic septic arthritis, as the longer the infection is present, the greater the accumulation of fibrin in the joint and the more severe the synovitis, meaning that the horse does not respond well to the process of joint lavage using needles alone (SCHNEIDER, 1998).

Oliveira (2008) states that another treatment option is to wash the joint, either with saline solution or 0.1% povidine-iodine. This method facilitates the resolution of the infection by removing harmful substances from the cartilage. The purulent effusion present in the joint slows down the action of many antibiotics, causing the pH to become acidic and interfering with the activity of aminoglycosides in particular (BAXTER; TURNER, 2006).

This procedure is an alternative to not having to perform arthroscopy, is more economically viable and does not require inducing the animal with general anaesthesia. In addition, joint lavage can be repeated several times during the treatment period, reducing the deleterious effects of the inflammatory response and removing inflammatory mediators from the joint space (MILNER et al., 2014; SANCHEZ-TERAN et al., 2016).

Another method widely used in horses with an infectious process in the distal portions of the limbs is intravenous regional perfusion. This technique ensures the accumulation of high concentrations of an antimicrobial in the synovial structures, soft tissues and bones (GODFREY; HARDY; COHEN, 2016).

Medication options include the use of corticosteroids, which act as an anti-inflammatory agent. Among the most common are triamcinolone, methylprednisolone and betamethasone, which act by inhibiting prostaglandin and phospholipase A2 synthesis. In addition, these drugs reduce the number and activity of neutrophils in the joint (MCCOY, 2017).

In addition to inhibiting the expression of collagenase genes (HUNTER; BLYTH, 1999), triamcinolone has been shown in experiments, along with betamethasone, to be one of the corticosteroids that has the least deleterious effect on articular cartilage. However, triamcinolone has a shorter duration in the body than betamethasone, and can be detected in the bloodstream up to seven days after administration (MCMURRAY, 2016), and should not exceed 18 mg per horse, as this can result in laminitis (BENTZ, 2015). The selection of antibiotics to be used should be based on the results of the culture and antibiogram. The most commonly used antimicrobial in regional infusions is amikacin, as it is less susceptible to inactivation by bacterial enzymes compared to other aminoglycosides. It reaches its peak concentration one hour after administration, with a half-life of five hours in foals and a minimum inhibitory concentration (MIC) of 16 iig/mL (DOWLING, 2004).

The MIC is a determining factor in the success of treatments for orthopaedic infections, and it is ideal to use concentrations above it (LEVINE et al., 2010). In the case of amikacin sulphate, the dosage during the regional perfusion procedure in horses can vary from 500 mg to 2.5 g diluted in 40-100 mL of 0.9% sodium chloride. It provides continuous suppression of bacterial growth after it has been exposed to the antibiotic (HARVEY et al., 2016) and reaches high concentrations in the synovial fluid (FIRTH et al., 1988).

To carry out this procedure in the tarsal region, the antibiotic of choice is administered into the medial saphenous vein (CIMETTI; MERRIAM; D'OENCH, 2004). To do this, the area is prepared aseptically, the animal is sedated and the needle or catheter is inserted into the vein with a syringe (HYDE et al., 2013) and a tourniquet is placed to occlude the superficial vascularisation, which is maintained for approximately thirty minutes. The antibiotic is injected into the portion of the vein located distal to the tourniquet (Figure 18), and the ideal volume is still unknown (RUBIO-MARTÍNEZ; CRUZ, 2006).

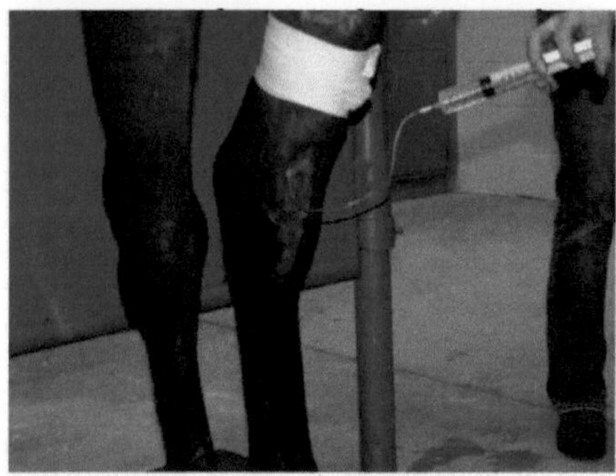

Figure 18 - Intravenous regional perfusion in the tarsal region of the left hind limb of a horse
Source: Rothenbuhlern, 2017.

Another form of treatment that is widely used in horses with septic arthritis is intra-articular injections. This technique is based on injecting different types of medication into the joint affected by joint disease (FERRIS et al., 2011).

According to Gillespie, Adams and Moore (2016), the site needs to be cleaned with an antiseptic, such as 2% chlorhexidine, which may or may not be after trichotomy. A local anaesthetic is then used to administer the antibiotic of choice, of which amikacin and gentamicin are the two most commonly used.

Hyaluronic acid and/or corticosteroids can also be used (LINDHOLM et al., 2002), respecting the correct concentration, since if it is high, it can have an unfavourable influence on the structural organisation of collagens in the cartilage and inhibit the synthesis of proteoglycans (CARON, 2005).

Systemic antibiotic therapy is of great importance and must be carried out concomitantly with the treatments already described. Enrofloxacin is widely used when the administration period is long (5.5 mg/kg intravenously), but it is not used in foals as it can cause lesions in the hyaline cartilage (FERNANDES, 2012).

However, tetracycline derivatives can be administered to foals, such as doxycycline. It can be administered orally at a dose of 10 mg/kg every 12 hours, with a plasma concentration of 0.5 µg/niL. which is higher than the MIC, and can be detected in the aqueous humour, peritoneal fluid, endometrial tissue and synovial fluid, where elimination is slow and remains for approximately 72 hours after administration (SCHNABEL et al., 2010).

Non-steroidal anti-inflammatory drugs are also widely used to treat pain and inflammation in horses. Among the most commonly used are phenylbutazone (4 mg/kg), which acts on the affected joint and increases the use of the affected limb (SCHNEIDER, 1998) and flunixin meglumine, which has an analgesic action within two hours of application and lasts for approximately 36 hours, with the recommended dose being 0.25-1.1 mg/kg (STANLEY; KNYCH; LACK, 2017).

Firocoxib has shown promise in therapy for foals, as it has very low toxicity. It can be administered orally, which prevents repeated doses by injection and is easier to administer. It has a great analgesic and anti-inflammatory effect because it is a cyclooxygenase 2 (COX-2) inhibitor, and is as effective as phenylbutazone. It can be detected in synovial fluid and its half-life is five to ten times longer than that reported for other non-steroidal anti-inflammatory drugs, but it is not detected in plasma 72 hours after administration (HOVANESSIAN, 2012).

The use of anti-inflammatory drugs can cause gastrointestinal ulceration in foals, which is a major concern, especially between one week and six months of age (GEOR; PAPICH; ROUSSEAUX, 1989). It is very necessary to administer gastric protectors such as ranitidine, which, when administered orally, has a dose of 4.4 mg/Kg and is more bioavailable in foals than in adult horses (HOLLAND et al., 1997).

2.2.7 **Prognosis**

The prognosis depends on the number of joints affected, the extent of the bone lesion and the time that has passed since the infection began (MEIJER; WEEREN;

RIJKENHUIZEN, 2000). If the infection is controlled early, the prognosis can be very good, but usually in foals it can be worse than in adult horses, because there is often multiple organ involvement and septicaemia (MACDONALD et al., 2006). In these cases, whether due to economic factors, failure to respond to treatment, worsening clinical signs or lack of improvement, euthanasia is recommended (WRIGHT et al., 2016).

In chronic cases, when the patient undergoes arthroscopy, they can recover within 10 days, and the response to treatment is visible within 24 hours of the procedure. However, the rehabilitation time will depend on the affected joint, where for example, in the carpal region this can occur between 7-10 days and in the tibiotarsal joint in approximately 5 weeks (SCHNEIDER, 1998). The prognosis can also be poor if the disease is chronic and Gram-negative bacteria have been found to be more prevalent in these animals, often resulting in mortality (VOS; DUCHARME, 2008; QUINN et al., 2011).

According to Oliver et al. (2017), 78% of foals confirmed with septic arthritis survive the condition, indicating that the survival rate has increased over the years, especially if treatment is started within the first 24 hours. If this time is longer, the survival rate drops from 93 per cent to 66 per cent. The patient can be discharged within 6-37 days in acute cases, varying mainly according to the number of joints involved, but the prognosis is usually favourable.

2.2.8 **Prophylaxis**

Methods such as good handling practices, adopting measures in order to reduce the chances of sepsis in foals, endoscope-guided surgery immediately after trauma in order to prevent the contaminated joint from becoming an infected joint and manipulation of the joint, whatever it may be, should be done by aseptic procedure (ADAMS, 2017).

Prophylaxis through the administration of antibiotics is still necessary, but care must be taken to ensure that these drugs are used incorrectly, avoiding the development of antimicrobial resistance (BORG; CARMALT, 2013).

CHAPTER 3

CASE REPORT

3.1 HISTORY

A fifty-three-day-old male foal weighing 30kg and of no defined breed was treated at the UNIFESO Veterinary Medicine School Clinic in Teresópolis on 25/02/2016.

The animal was found by its guardian a few hours after birth with a barbed wire wrapped around the tarsal region of the right hind limb (RHL) and a laceration in the same area. According to the owner, in the days following the trauma there was an increase in volume at the site and a yellowish secretion draining from the wound. The foal was medicated with flunixin meglumine and penicillin (dose not reported) for a period of five days. During the period when there was discharge from the wound, the animal was able to support its limb on the ground. However, after healing, there was no more secretion, there was a pronounced enlargement of the area and the foal began to show progressive lameness of the affected limb. The owner reported that during this period, the foal showed active behaviour and suckled regularly. There was no veterinary care prior to the consultation at UNIFESO. The medication administered was done so without a veterinary prescription. Data on colostrum quality and intake is unknown, as is the mare's vaccination and deworming history.

3.2 CLINICAL FOLLOW-UP

At the animal's first appointment, held on 25/02/2016, the foal was identified and given an anamnesis. During the physical examination, the patient had normal-coloured mucous membranes, with a capillary refill time of less than three seconds; normal skin turgor; normal digestive auscultation, as well as respiratory and cardiac auscultation without abnormalities and within normal parameters. Feeding was normal and, according to the tutor, the mare was breastfeeding regularly.

On inspection, it was possible to see that there was a scar and oedema in the region of the right tarsus, and that the limb could only be supported by forceps. Palpation revealed that the oedema was rigid and there was heat in the area. During passive flexion of the limb, the animal showed no pain, but there was reduced movement of the joint. The animal was then examined while walking and trotting on a hard surface, where grade 4 claudication was found (without the limb resting on the ground and with strong head movement) according to AAEP.There was no sign of crepitus, which intensified the suspicion of a possible infection and local inflammation, suggestive of traumatic septic arthritis. At the same time, there was hyperextension of the fetlock of the left hind limb, due to the increased weight on it.

On the same day, the animal underwent X-ray examination of the tibio-tarsal and tarso-metatarsal regions of the MPD in the dorsoplantar (DP) position of the tarsus (Figure 19.A); lateral position of the tarsus (Figure 19.B); dorsolateral plantar-medial oblique (DLPMO) position of the tarsus (Figure 19.C) and dorsolateral plantar-medial oblique (DMPLO) position of the tarsus (Figure 19.D).Radiographic findings indicated the presence of subchondral bone sclerosis, a decrease in joint space, loss of trabecular pattern in the distal third of the tibia, periarticular oedema, increased soft tissue opacity adjacent to the tibiotarsal joint, periosteal proliferation and alteration of the joint surface.

It was decided to perform a tibiotarsal arthrocentesis and the animal was taken to the operating theatre and placed on the operating table, where it was restrained without the need for sedation. The site was previously trichotomised and antiseptically cleaned. Arthrocentesis was carried out on the medial side of the limb with a 30x8 needle, taking care not to hit the saphenous vein, which was introduced distally to the medial malleolus of the tibia. However, this was unsuccessful, as there was no synovial fluid available to be collected. Taking into account the history and clinical examination, the decision was made to apply amikacin (250 mg) and triamcinolone (2 mg) intra-articularly, these being the total doses per joint.Flunixin meglumine (1.1 mg/kg) was prescribed orally (VO) for five days and doxycycline (10 mg/kg) twice a day for seven days, VO. As there were no changes in the physical parameters suggestive of systemic disease, and due to financial restrictions, it was decided not to carry out a blood count, and the foal was released after the procedure. The animal's guardian was asked to return to the clinic after seven days for a new assessment and follow-up of the patient.

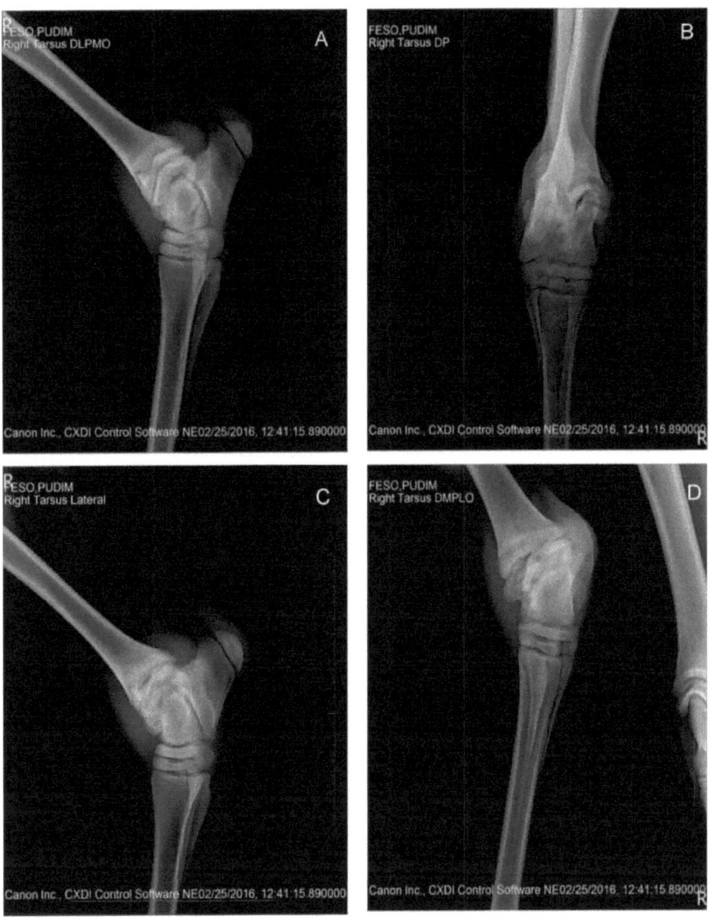

Figure 19 - Dorsoplantar (A), lateral (B), dorsolateral (C) and dorsomedial (D) views of the tarsus, showing reduced joint space, sclerosis of subchondral bone, loss of trabecular pattern in the tibia, periarticular oedema, periosteal proliferation, altered joint surface and increased soft tissue opacity.
Source: Author

At the second appointment, held on 03/03/2016, the foal weighed 32kg, was active and neighed. According to the owner, breastfeeding was normal, the animal didn't lie down for long, it moved around a lot despite its condition and always tried to be close to its mother. There were no changes in vital parameters compared to the previous examination.

On inspection of the MPD, it was still resting on the clamp. On palpation, there was a reduction in oedema in the tarsal region and a slight increase in joint mobility.

The patient was taken to the operating theatre for regional perfusion of the affected area, by making a tourniquet proximal to the area which was perfused with amikacin (250 mg) diluted in 20 mL of saline solution. With the saphenous vein engorged, lidocaine was applied around it to ensure local anaesthesia, and then accessed with a number 22 scalpel through which the medication was applied slowly. The tourniquet was kept on for thirty minutes to ensure that the antibiotic penetrated the joints

At the end of the procedure, firocoxib (0.1 mg/kg) in oral solution was prescribed, to be administered once a day for seven days and doxycycline (10mg/kg) was continued twice a day for seven days, VO. The tutor was recommended to design footwear for the MPD so that the foal could support the limb on the ground and reduce the contraction of the superficial and deep flexor tendons, while also avoiding overloading the left posterior, as this was receiving a greater load than normal.

Once again, the animal was asked to return to the clinic in seven days for a new assessment, follow-up and continuation of treatment.

At the third appointment, held on 10/03/2016, the foal showed active behaviour, no signs of lethargy, weighed 34 kg and was breastfeeding regularly. During the general physical examination, there were no changes in vital parameters compared to the previous examination. In the specific physical examination of the locomotor system, the patient continued not to support the MPD on the ground, the oedema in the region of the right tarsus had reduced considerably, in passive flexion no pain points were observed, although there was still a reduction in joint mobility and during palpation of the site no increase in temperature was detected, as was identified on the first day. The angulation of the MEP fetlock was more flattened. The patient underwent a new process of regional perfusion of the right tarsus, as described above, with the area perfused with amikacin (250 mg/joint) diluted in 20 mL of physiological solution.

The animal's guardian reported that he hadn't had any success with the idealised footwear, as had been suggested during the previous consultation, saying that the foal wouldn't support his limb on the ground and raised it even higher. They decided to make a new one, using wood that was sawn into the shape of the hoof and fixed to it using a bandage and adhesive plaster, as can be seen in figures 20 A and B.

He was then asked to maintain the previously prescribed medication, firocoxib (0.1mg/kg) in oral solution, once a day and doxycycline (10mg/kg) twice a day VO and to return within a week for a new assessment.

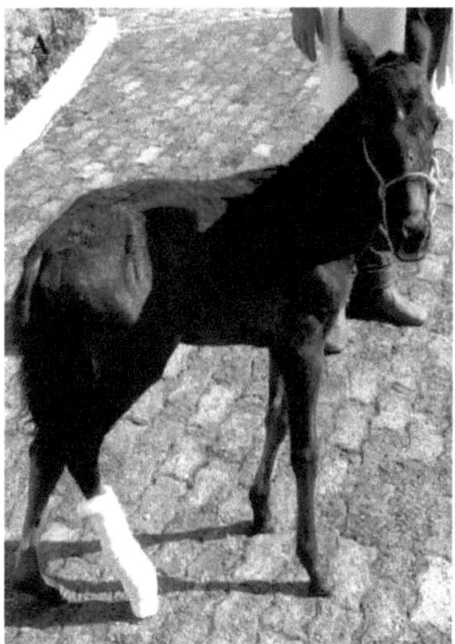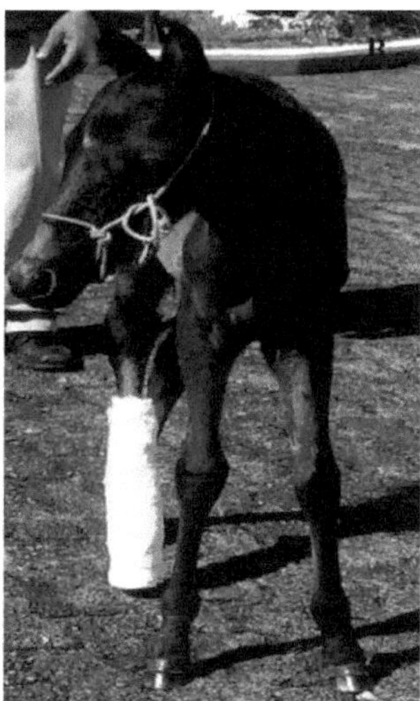

Figure 20: Foal in lateral (A) and frontal (B) view with shoes and bandage on the right hind limb
Source: Own authorship.

At the fourth appointment, held on 17/03/2016, during the general physical assessment, the foal showed no abnormalities when compared to the previous days' appointments, and was alert, active, weighing 37kg, moving around, with an appetite and regular breastfeeding, and had no systemic alterations. The general physical examination showed no changes in vital parameters compared to the previous examination.

During a specific physical test of the locomotor system, it was noted that the affected limb was still not supported on the floor, even though it was wearing shoes, and was more contracted than it had been the previous week. There was no oedema in the tarsal region or pain on palpation and no increase in local temperature.

The patient had a progressive degree of flattening of the MEP, especially as he was growing and consequently increasing in weight.

The animal underwent a new process of regional perfusion of the right tarsus, as described above, with the area perfused with amikacin (250 mg/joint) diluted in 20 mL of physiological solution.

Flunixin meglumine (1.1 mg/ kg) was prescribed to be administered once a day for five days via IM and ranitidine hydrochloride (0.5 mg/kg) twice a day for six days, VO.

The guardian was asked to bring the patient back after a week for another consultation and an X-ray of the hip joint, as the reason for the limb not being supported and elevated could have a more upward origin.

At the fifth consultation, held on 23-03-2016, the patient weighed 37 kg and showed behavioural changes, being apathetic and lethargic. According to his guardian, he appeared to be more tired, had greater difficulty moving around and spent most of the day lying down. General physical examinations were no different from the previous week, with a heart rate of around 114 beats per minute (bpm). The temperature was measured transrectally and was high, at around 39.4, but this was justifiable given that the foal was transported in a utility vehicle and kept in the sun while waiting for the service.

The specific physical examination of the locomotor system didn't reveal much difference when compared to the previous results, apart from the suspension of the MPD which was on a larger scale, increasing the height difference between the limb and the floor.

Due to the lack of clinical progress and in order to prevent the animal from suffering, the guardian and the veterinary team involved in the case decided that the most advisable procedure would be to euthanise the patient, signing an authorisation form to carry out the procedure and donating the corpse for *post-mortem* analysis.

The foal was euthanised, humanely induced with xylazine and thiopental, and intravenously administered potassium chloride. In the Animal Clinical Pathology laboratory, the foal's MPD was assessed *post-mortem to* check for anomalies in the tarsal joints. The limb was dissected at the tibio-tarsal joint, where the skin and muscles were first removed and then the internal region of the joint was accessed using a scalpel. The analysis revealed the presence of a loss of joint capsule, part of the tendon of the cranial tibial muscle (cuneus tendon) was adherent, the synovial pouch underneath was dry and showing signs of fibrosis, proliferation of fibrous tissue, loss of movement in the joint due to an ankylosing process, loss of synovial membrane and absence of synovial fluid, as shown in figure 21 A and B.

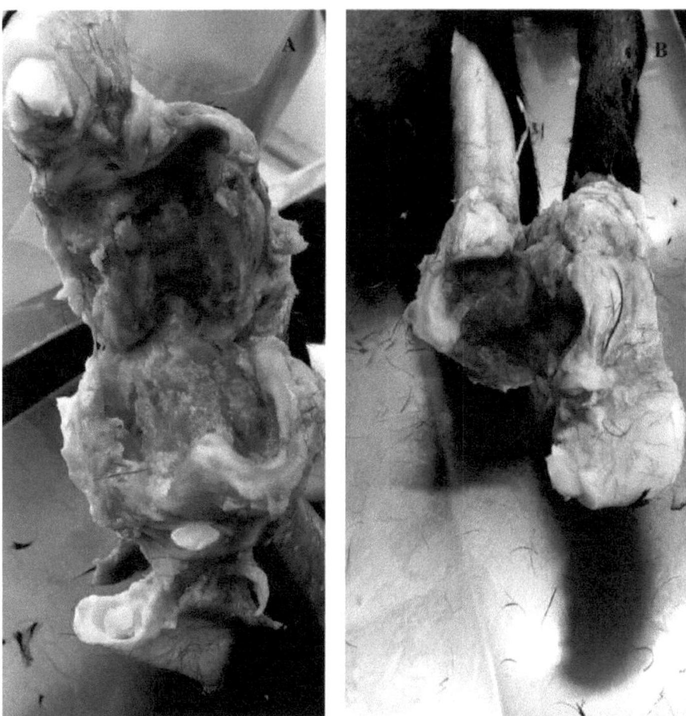

Figura 21   A and B- Erosive process of the tibiotarsal articular surface with consequent loss of structures

Source: Own authorship.

CHAPTER 4

DISCUSSION

The presence of a yellowish secretion draining from the wound in the tarsal region, days after the incident, supposedly indicated a process of infection, possibly due to the presence of bacteria in the joint, in agreement with Shirtliff and Mader (2002). These microorganisms may have gained access to the joint after the trauma occurred, as described by Hiber and Darling (2012).

We observed weeks after the accident, in addition to the MPD's lameness, oedema in the affected area resulting from the non-drainage of the secretion produced after healing, which is in line with the symptoms presented in animals with septic arthritis according to Rizzoni and Miyauchi (2012).

During the clinical examination, the animal did not show any signs of systemic disease, but only local alterations caused by the laceration. Although the quality and intake of the colostrum was not assessed, the foal showed no signs of systemic infection at any time during its visits to the School Clinic. Therefore, with the existence of the sharp trauma in the tarsal region, the hypothesis of haematogenous septic arthritis was ruled out, which is in line with what Glass and Watts (2017) described, since they justify haematogenous septic arthritis by the existence of a failure in the passive transfer of antibodies, respiratory tract disorders, umbilical diseases or gastrointestinal infections and signs of septicaemia, which in the case of the patient in question these signs were not present.

As a way of improving the diagnosis, an attempt was made to collect synovial fluid by arthrocentesis, in agreement with Glass and Watts (2017), who report that this assessment is extremely important in cases of septic arthritis. However, this was unsuccessful, as there was no synovial fluid in the joint, in agreement with Baxter (2008), who explains that when the course of the infection is long-lasting, there is a high probability of permanent damage to the synovial structure and abnormalities in the articular cartilage.

Another auxiliary diagnostic method was radiography, which showed the presence of subchondral bone sclerosis, a decrease in joint space, loss of trabecular pattern in the distal third of the tibia, periarticular oedema, increased soft tissue opacity adjacent to the tibiotarsal joint, periosteal proliferation and altered joint surface. These findings are consistent with the damage caused by septic arthritis, as observed by Vieira (2009), Mostafa; Abu-Seida and El-Glil (2014) and Shirtliff and Mader (2002), although the loss of the trabecular pattern is not mentioned by these authors.

The changes found on the X-ray are probably the result of degenerative damage associated with the inflammatory and infectious process in the joint, which is in line with Ludwig et al. (2016).

For the treatment, we opted for intra-articular injection with amikacin and triamcinolone and regional perfusion using amikacin, which agrees with Hunter and Blyth (1999) and Mcmurray (2016) who report the use of this corticosteroid as a choleganase inhibitor, with a prolonged duration of seven days, generating the least possible deleterious effect on the articular cartilage. As it wasn't possible to collect the synovial fluid for culture, we opted to use amikacin, as it is one of the least susceptible to inactivation by bacterial enzymes among the existing aminoglycosides and has a better antimicrobial effect, making it the antibiotic of choice in this case, as explained by Dowling (2004).

The anti-inflammatory flunixin meglumine was chosen because it has analgesic action from two hours after administration and its effect lasts for approximately 36 hours, according to Stanley, Knych and Lack (2017). Firocoxib was chosen because it has good results during treatment in foals, has low toxicity, has an analgesic effect and is also an anti-inflammatory, as highlighted by Hovanessian (2012). Among the existing antibiotics, doxycycline was chosen because it can be administered orally and has a long half-life of approximately 72 hours, as defined by Schnabel et al. (2010).

The use of ranitidine was adopted as a preventative for gastrointestinal ulcers, as it has a higher bioavailability in foals than in adult horses, making it advisable for the case reported, in line with HOLLAND et al. (1997).

Because the animal was not treated correctly immediately after the trauma, the progression of septic arthritis resulted in complex damage to the foal's joint and irreversible damage to the articular cartilage. This process is in line with Schneider's (1998) explanation that the longer the infection is present, the greater the accumulation of fibrin in the joint and the more severe the synovitis, making it more difficult to respond to treatment. The patient's articular cartilage was degraded, confirming Baxter's (2008) report that once destroyed, the damage to the articular cartilage cannot be reversed, characterising the final stage of septic arthritis, contributing to the impediment of the joint's anatomical function.

The clinical changes in the foal's joints were unrecoverable and did not respond to treatment. It was decided to euthanise the animal, as the conditions were incompatible with the life of an equine, which over time would increase in weight and would not be able to stand on three legs, not guaranteeing the patient's well-being, in agreement with Wright et al. (2016) who confirm that when there is a failure to respond to treatment, worsening of clinical signs or if there is no improvement, euthanasia is the most appropriate course of action.

CHAPTER 5

FINAL CONSIDERATIONS

Despite the treatment adopted, the alterations generated by the initial injury to the hock could not be reversed, since there was complete destruction of the joint environment, due to the chronicity of the septic arthritis, possibly resulting from the lack of early treatment, which culminated in a worsening of the patient's clinical condition.

As the foal got older and its body weight increased, supporting it on three limbs became incompatible with the animal's well-being.

The lack of a positive response to the treatment adopted led to euthanasia as the final decision.

CHAPTER 6

REFERENCES

ABDELNOUR, A.; ARVIDSON, S.; BREMELL, T.; RYDÉN, C.; TARKOWSKI,
A. The accessory gene regulator (agr) controls *Staphylococcus aureus* virulence in a
murine arthritis model. **Infection and Immunity**, v. 61, n. 9, p. 3879-3885, 1993.

ADAMS, S. B. **Therapy for septic joints in the horse**. Available at:
<http://c.ymcdn.com/sites/www.invma.org/resource/resmgr/imported/SepticArthritis
1.pdf>. Accessed on: 27 August 2017.

ALVES, A. L. G. Semiology of the equine locomotor system. In: FEITOSA, F. L. F.
Semiologia veterinária - A arte do diagnóstico. 2. ed. São Paulo: ROCA, 2008.
p.569 -609.

ANNEAR, M. J.; FURR, M. O.; WHITE, N. A. Septic arthritis in foals. **Equine
Veterinary Education**, v. 23, n. 8, p. 422-431, 2011.
Arthritis. **American Association of Equine Practitioners**, v. 52, p. 5-12, 2006.

BARBER, S. Management of wounds of the neck and body. In: STASHAK, T. S.;
THEORET, C. L. **Equine wound management.** 2.ed. Singapore: Wiley-Blackwell,
2008. p. 333-372.

BAXTER, G. M. Diagnosis and Management of wounds involving synovial
structures. In: STASHAK, T. S.; THEORET, C. L. **Equine Wound Management**.
2.ed. Singapore: Blackwell, 2008. p. 463 - 468.

BAXTER, G. M.; TURNER, A. S. Bone diseases and related structures. In:
STASHAK, T. S. **Claudication in horses according to Adams'**. 5. ed. São Paulo:
Roca, 2006. p.363 - 401.

BECCATI, F.; GIALLETTI, R.; PASSAMONTI, F.; NANNARONE, S.; MEO, A.
D.; PEPE, M. Ultrasonographic findings in 38 horses with septic arthritis/tenosyvitis.
Veterinary Radiology and Ultrasound, v. 56, n. 1, p. 68-76, 2015.

BENTZ, B. Clinical pharmacology of the equine musculoskeletal system. In: COLE,
C.; BENTZ, B.; MAXWELL, L. Equine pharmacology. India: Wiley Blackwell,
2015. p. 218-253.

BODAAN, C. J.; RILEY, C. B.; ENGELI, E. **Evaluation of a caudolateral
approach for arthrocentesis and injection of the equine elbow joint.** Available at:
< http://veterinaryrecord.bmj.com/content/early/2016/06/16/vr.103738.info>.
Accessed on: 08 August 2017.

BORG, H.; CARMALT, J. L. Postoperative septic arthritis after elective equine arthroscopy without antimicrobial prophylaxis. **Veterinary Surgery**, v. 42, n. 3, p. 262-266, 2013.

CABLE, C. S. **Septic arthritis: joint savings**. Available at: <http://www.thehorse.com/articles/10023/septic-arthritis-joint-savings>. Accessed on: 16 August 2017.

CARON, J. P. Intra articular injections for joint disease in horses. **Veterinary Clinics Equine Practice**, v. 21, n. 3, p. 559-573, 2005.

CARON, J. P. Osteoarthritis. In: ROSS, M. W.; DYSON, S. J. **Diagnosis and management of lameness in the horse.** 1.ed. Missouri: Saunders, 2003. p. 572-591.

CARTER, G. K. Infectious joint disease. In: COLAHAN, P. T.; MAYHEW, I. G.; MERRITT, A. M.; MOORE, J. N. **Equine medicine and surgery**. 4.ed. v.II. United States of America: American Veterinary Publications, INC, 1991. p. 14771478.

CIMETTI, L. J.; MERRIAM, J. G.; D'OENCH, S. N. How to perform intravenous regional limb perfusion using amikacin and DMSO. In: **Annual Convention of the American Association of Equine Practitioners**, 50, 2004. Denver, Colorado: P1429.1204 Ithaca, NY: International Veterinary Information Service, 2004. p. 219223.

COSTA, M. H. C. G. da. **Incidence of locomotor injuries in horses diagnosed by x-ray.** 2012. 84f. Dissertation (Master's in Veterinary Medicine), Lusófona University of Humanities and Technology, 2012.

DENG, G. M.; TARKOWSKI, A. The features of arthritis induced by cpg motifs in bacterial DNA. **Arthritis and Rheumatism**, v. 43, n. 2, p. 356-364, 2000.

DOWLING, P. M. Antimicrobial therapy. In: BERTONE, J. J.; HORSPOOL, L. J. I. **Equine clinical pharmacology.** China: ELSEVIER, p. 13-47, 2004.

DURHAM, M.; DYSON, S. J. Applied anatomy of the musculoskeletal system. In: ROSS, M. W.; DYSON, S. J. **Diagnosis and management of lameness in the horse.** 1.ed. Missouri: Elsevier, 2003. p. 81-93.

DYCE, K. M.; SACK, W. O.; WENSING, C. J. G. **Treatise on veterinary anatomy**. 4. ed. Rio de Janeiro: Elsevier, 2010. p. 624-643.

EASLEY, J. T.; BROKKEN, M. T.; ZUBROD, B. C.; MORTON, A. J.; GARRETT, K. S.; HOLMES, S. P. Magnetic resonance imaging findings in horses with septic arthritis. **Veterinary Radiology and Ultrasound**, v. 52, n. 4, p. 402-408, 2011.

FERNANDES, A. C. E. G. **Penetrating wounds to the sole and groin caused by sharp objects**. 2012. 51f. Dissertation (Integrated Master's Degree in Veterinary Medicine), University of Porto, 2012.

FERRIS, D. J.; FRISBIE, D. D.; MCILWRAITH, C. W.; KAWCAK, C. E. Current joint therapy usage in equine practice: A survey of veterinarians 2009. **Equine Veterinary Journal**, v. 45, n. 5, p. 530-535, 2011.

FIRTH, E. C.; KLEIN, W. R.; NOUWS, F. M.; WESING, T. Effect of induced synovial inflammation on pharmacokinetics and synovial concentration of sodium ampicillin and kanamycin sulfate after systemic administration in ponies. **Journal of Veterinary Pharmacology and Therapeutics**, v. 11, n. 1, p. 56-62, 1988.

FISCHER, A. T.; HARDY, J.; LÉVEILLÉ, R.; RIJKENHUIZEN, A. B. M.; AUER, J. A. Minimally invasive surgical techniques. In: AUER, J. A.; STICK, J. A. **Equine Surgery.** 3.ed. United States of America: Saunders, 2006. p. 161-170.

FONSECA, F. A.; ZAMBRANO, R. S.; DIAS, G. M. B.; LIMA, E. M. M.; ALVES, G. E. S.; GODOY, R. F. Physicochemical and cytological characteristics of temporomandibular joint synovial fluid in horses. **Pesquisa Veterinária Brasileira**, v. 29, n. 10, p. 829-833, 2009.

FRISBIE D. D. Synovial joint biology and pathhobiology. In: AUER, J. A.; STICK, J.A. **Equine Surgery.**4.ed. Philadelphia: Elsevier, 2012. p. 1096-1114.

GALLO, M. A. **Study of the incidence of osteochondrosis dissecans in the tibiotarsal joint of three-year-old horses (Equus caballos) of the Brazilian Equestrian breed in the state of São Paulo, using digital field radiography.** 2010. 52f. Dissertation (Master's Degree in Veterinary Surgical Medicine) - Faculty of Veterinary Medicine and Zootechny, University of São Paulo, 2010.

GASCHEN, L., LEROUX, A.; TRICHEL, J.; RIGGS, L.; BRAGULLA, H. H.; RADEMACHER, N.; RODRIUEZ, D. Magnetic resonance imaging in foals with infectious arthritis. Veterinary Radiology and Ultrasound, v. 52, n. 6, p. 627-633, 2011.

GEOR, R. J.; PAPICH, M. G.; ROUSSEAUX, C. The protective effects of sulcralfate and ranitidine in foals experimentally intoxicated with phenylbutazone. Canadian Journal of Veterinary Research, v. 53, n. 2, p. 231-238, 1989.

GETTY, R. **Anatomy of Domestic Animals**. v. 1, 5.ed. Rio de Janeiro: Guanabara Koogan, 1986. 1134 p.

GILLESPIE, C. C.; ADAMS, S. B.; MOORE, G. E. Methods and variables associated with the risk of septic arthritis following intra-articular injections in horses: A survey of veterianrians. **Veterinary Surgery**, v.45, n. 8, p. 1071-1076, 2016.

GJERTSSON, I.; JONSSON, I. M.; PESCHEL, A.; TARKOWSKI, A.; LINDHOLM, C. Formylated peptides are important virulence factors in *Staphylococcus aureus* arthritis in mice. **The Journal of Infectious Diseases**, v. 205, n. 2, p. 305-311, 2012.

GLASS, K.; WATTS, A. E. Septic arthritis, physitis, and osteomyelitis in foals. **Veterinary Clinic Equine**, v.33, n.2, p. 299-314, 2017.

GODFREY, J. L.; HARDY, J.; COHEN, N. D. Effects of regional limb perfusion volume on concentrations of amikacin sulfate in synovial and interstitial fluid samples from anesthetised horses. **American Journal of Veterinary Research**, v. 77, n. 6, p. 582-588, 2016.

GRAUW, J. C. de.; DONABÉDIAN, M.; LEST, C. H. A. d.; PERONA, G.; ROBERT, C.; LEPAGE, O.; ROSSET, W. M.; WEEREN, P. R. van. Assessment of synovial fluid biomarkers in healthy foals and in foals with tarsocrural osteochondrosis. **The Veterinary Journal**, v. 190, n. 3, p. 390-395, 2011.

HARDY, J. Etiology, diagnosis, and treatment of septic arthritis, osteitis, and osteomyelitis in foals. **Clinic Technique Equine**, v. 5, p. 309-317, 2006.

HARVEY, A.; KILCOYNE, I.; BYRNE, B. A.; NIETO, J. Effect of dose on intraarticular amikacin sulfate concentrations following intravenous regional limb perfusion in horses. **Veterinary Surgery**, v. 45, n. 8, p. 1077-1082 , 2016.

HIBER, L.; DARLING, K. T. Zoonotic diseases. In: CAVENEY, L.; JONES, B.; ELLIS, K. **Veterinary infection prevention and control**. New Delhi: Wiley-Blackwell, 2012. p. 75-76.

HOLLAND, P. S.; BRUMBAUGH, G. W.; RUOFF, W. W.; BROWN, S. A. Plasma pharmacokinetics of ranitidine HCL in foals. **Journal of Veterinary Pharmacology Therapy**, v. 20, n. 6, p. 447-452, 1997.

HOVANESSIAN, N. **The pharmacokinetics of firocoxib after multiple oral doses to neonatal foals**. 2012. 65f. Dissertation (Master's Degree in Biomedical and Veterinary Sciences) - Virginia Polytechnic Institute and State University, 2012.

HUNTER, J. A.; BLYTH, T. H. A risk-benefit assessment of intra-articular corticosteroids in rheumatic disorders. Drug Safety, v. 21, n. 5, p. 353- 365, 1999.

HYDE, R. M.; LYNCH, T. M.; CLARK, C. K.; SLONE, D. E.; HUGHES, F. E. The influence of perfusate volume on antimicrobial concentration in synovial fluid following intravenous regional limb perfusion in the standing horse. **Canadian Veterinary Journal**, v. 54, n. 4, p. 363-367, 2013.

JACKMAN, B. R. Review of equine distal hock inflammation and arthritis. **American Association of Equine Practioners**, v. 52, p. 5-12, 2006.

JACOBSEN, S.; THOMSEN, M. H.; NANNI, S. Concentrations of serum amyloid A in serum and synovial fluid from healthy horses and horses with joint disease. **American Journal of Veterinary Research**, v. 67, n. 10, p. 1738-1742, 2006.

KAINER, R. A. Functional anatomy of the locomotor system. In: STASHAK, T. S.

Claudication in horses according to Adams'. 5.ed. São Paulo: Roca, 2006. p.1 - 53.

KAWCAK, C. Biomechanics in Joint. In: MCILWRAITH, C. W.; FRISBIE, D. D.; KAWCAK, C.; WEEREN, R. V. Joint disease in the horse. 2.ed. China: Elsevier, 2016. p. 25-30.

LEVINE, D. G.; EPSTEIN, K. L.; AHERN, B. J.; RICHARDSON, D. W. Efficacy of three tourniquet types for intravenous antimicrobial regional limb perfusion in standing horses. **Veterinary Surgery**, v. 39, n. 8, p. 1021-1024, 2010.

LINDHOLM, A. C.; SWENSSON, U.; MITRI, N. de.; COLLINDER, E. Clinical effects of betamethasone and hyaluronan, and of defocalised carbon dioxide laser treatment on traumatic arthritis in the fetlock joints of horses. **Journal of Veterinary Medicine**, v. 49, n.4, p. 189-194, 2002.

LUDWIG, E. K.; WIESE, R. B.; GRAHAM, M. R.; TYLER, A. J.; SETTLAGE, J. M.; WERE, S. R.; WOLFE, C. S. P.; MULLARKY, I. K.; DAHLGREN, L. A. Serum and synovial fluid serum amyloid a response in equine models of synovitis and septic arthritis. **Veterinary Surgery**, v. 45, n. 7, p. 859-867, 2016.

MACDONALD, M. H.; KANNEGIETER, N.; PERONI, J. F.; MERFY, W. E. The musculoskeletal system. In: HIGGINS, A. J.; SNYDER, J. R. The equine manual. 2.ed. China: Elsevier, 2006, p. 937-943.

MALCIUS, D.; JONKUS, M.; KUPRIONIS, G.; MALECKAS, A.; MONASTYRECKIENE, E.; UKTVERIS, R.; RINKEVICIUS, S.; BARAUSKAS, V. The accuracy of different imaging techniques in diagnosis of acute haematogenous osteomyelitis. Medicina, v. 45, n. 8, p. 624-631, 2009.

MCCOY, A. M. Recent advances in equine osteoarthritis. Available at: < https://www.isvma.org/wp-content/uploads/2016/10/RecentAdvancesinEquineOsteoarthritis.pdf>. Accessed on 12 August 2017.

MCILWRAITH, C. W. Disease processes of synovial membrane, fibrous capsule, ligaments, and articular cartilage. **American Association of Equine Practitioners**, v. 57, p. 142-156, 2001.

MCILWRAITH, C. W. Diseases of the joints, tendons, ligaments and related structures. In: STASHAK, T. S. **Claudication in horses according to Adam's**. 5.ed. São Paulo: Rocca, 2006. p. 417-597.

MCILWRAITH, C. W.; NIXON, A. J.; WRIGHT, I. M. **Diagnostic and surgical arthroscopy in the horse**. 4.ed. China: Elsevier, 2015. 454p.

MCMURRAY, J. Equine pathology and clinic. 2016. 102f. Dissertation (Integrated Master's Degree in Veterinary Medicine), University of Évora, 2016.

MEIJER, M. C.; WEEREN, P. R. V.; RIJKENHUIZEN, A. B. M. Clinical experiences of treating septic arthritis in the equine by repeated joint lavage: a series of 39 cases. **Journal Veterinary Medicine**, v. 47, n. 6, p. 351-365, 2000.

MILLER, G. **Hock pain is prevalent in horses: A horse's hock problems may begin years before they are noticed**. Available at: < http://horse-journal.com/article/hock-pain-is-prevalent-5175>. Accessed on: 01 Feb 2017.

MILNER, P. I.; BARDELL, D. A.; WARNER, L.; PACKER, M. J.; SENIOR, J. M.; SINGER, E. R.; ARCHER, D. C. Factors associated with survival to hospital discharge following endoscopic treatment for synovial sepsis in 214 horses. **Equine Veterinary Journal**, v. 46, n. 6, p. 701-705, 2014.

MOLLER, N. C. R.; WEEREN, P. R. V. How exercise influences equine joint homeostasis. **Veterinary Journal**, v. 222, p. 60-67, 2017.

MORTON, A. J. Diagnosis and treatment of septic arthritis. **Veterinary Clinic Equine**, v. 21, p. 627-649, 2005.

MOSTAFA, M. B.; ABU-SEIDA, A. M.; EL-GLIL, A. I. A. Septic tarsitis in horses: clinical, radiological, ultrasonographic, arthroscopic and bacteriological findings. Research Opinions in **Animal** and **Veterinary** Sciences, v. 4, n. 1, p. 30-34, 2014.

MOTTA, R.G., MARTINS, L. S. A. MOTTA, I. G., GUERRA, S. T., PAULA, C. L. de., BOLAMOS, C. A. D., SILVA, R. C. da., RIBEIRO, M. G. Multidrug resistant bacteria isolated from septic arthritis in horses. **Pesquisa Veterinária Brasileira,** v. 37, n. 4, p. 325-330, 2017.

NEUENSCHWANDER, H. M. **Comparison of the effects of intra-articular application of hyaluronic acid of different molecular weights in a model of acute synovitis induced by LPS in horses.** 2016. 82f. Dissertation (Master's in Veterinary Medicine) - Faculty of Veterinary Medicine and Zootechny, University of São Paulo, 2016.

OLIVER, F.B.; RUSSEL, T. M.; UPRICHARD, K. L.; NEIL, K. M.; POLLOCK, P. J. Treatment of septic arthritis of the coxofemoral joint in 12 foals. **Veterinary surgery**, v. 46, n. 4, p. 530-538, 2017.

OLIVEIRA, C. E. F. de. **Traumatic locomotor disorders in vaquero horses (Equus caballus, LINNAEUS, 1758) treated at the Veterinary Hospital /UFCG, Patos - PB**. 2008. 55f. Course Conclusion Paper (Veterinary Medicine Course) - Federal University of Campina Grande, Paraíba, 2008.

PALMEIRA, R.B. **Osteopathies in horses (Eqiiiis _caballus, Linnaeus,_ 1758) - casuistry at the veterinary hospital /cstr /ufcg, patos - pb.** 2008. 80f. Final Course Work (Veterinary Medicine Course) - Federal University of Campina Grande, Paraíba, 2008.

PALMQVIST, N.; SILVERMAN, G. J.; JOSEFSSON, E.; TARKOWSKI, A. Bacterial cell wall-expressed proteinA triggers supraclonal B-cell responses upon in vivo infection with *Staphylococcus aureus*. **Microbes and Infection**, v.7, n. 15, p. 1501-1511, 2005.

PARADIS, R. M. Manifestations of septicaemia. In: ______. **Equine neonatology: A case-based approach**. Hong Kong: Elsevier, 2006. p.112-120.

PORTER, E. G.; WERPY, N. M. New concepts in standing advanced diagnostic equine imaging. Veterinary Clinic Equine, v. 30, n. 1, p.239-268, 2014.

QUINN, P. J., MARKEY, B. K.; LEONARD, F. C., FITZPATRICK, E. S., FANNING, S., HARTIGAN, P. J. **Veterinary Microbiology and Microbial Disease**. 2.ed. Hong Kong: Wiley-Blackwell, 2011. 1231p.

RIJT, M. P. V. de. **Radiographic and echographic changes in osteoarthritis of the metacarpophalangeal joint in sport horses.** 2011. 85f. Dissertation (Master's in Veterinary Medicine) - Lusófona University of Humanities and Technologies, Lisbon, 2011.

RIZZONI, L. B.; MIYAUCHI, T. A. Main diseases of equine neonates. **Acta Veterinária Brasilica**, v. 6, n. 1, p. 9-16, 2012.

RUBIO-MARTÍNEZ, L. M.; CRUZ, A. M. Antimicrobial regional limb perfusion in horses. **Journal of the American Veterinary Medical Association**, v. 228, n. 5, p. 706-712, 2006.

SANCHEZ-TERAN, A. F.; BRACAMONTE, J. L.; HENRICK, S.; RIDDELL, L.; MUSIL, K.; HOFF, B.; MARTÍNEZ, L. M. R. Effect of repeated through-and-through joint lavage on serum amyloid A in synovial fluid from healthy horses. **The Veterinary Journal**, v. 210, p. 30-33, 2016.

SCANZELLO, C. R.; GOLDRING, S. R. The role of synovitis in osteoarthritis pathogenesis. **Bone**, v. 51, n. 2, p. 249-257, 2012.

SCHNABEL, L. V.; PAPICH, M. G.; WATTS, A. E.; FORTIER, L. A. Orally administered doxycycline accumulates in synovial fluid compared to plasma. Equine Veterinary Journal, v. 42, n. 3, p. 208-212, 2010.

SCHNEIDER, R. K. Synovial and osseous infections. In: AUER, J. A.; STICK, J. A. **Equine Surgery.** 3.ed. United States of America: Saunders, 2006. p.1121 - 1129.

SCHNEIDER, R. K. Treatment of posttraumatic septic arthritis. **American Association of Equine Practitioners,** v. 44, p. 167-171, 1998.

SCHNEIDER, R. K.; BRAMLAGE, L. R.; MOORE, R. M.; MECKLENBURG, L. M.; KOHN, C. W.; GABEL, A. A retrospective study of 192 horses affected with septic arthritis/tenosynovitis. **Equine Veterinary Journal**, v. 24, n. 6, p. 436-442, 1992.

SELLNOW, L. **Tendons and Ligaments: anatomy and physiology.** Available at: <

http://www.thehorse.com/articles/16765/tendons-and-ligaments-anatomy-and-physiology>. Accessed on: 05 August 2017.

SHIRTLIFF, M. E.; MADER, J. M. Acute septic arthritis. **Clinical Microbiology Reviews**, v. 15, n. 4, p. 527-544, 2002.

SOUZA, R. S. de.; PINHAL, M. A. S. **Interactions in physiological processes: the importance of the dynamics between extracellular matrix and proteoglycans.** Available at: < http://files.bvs.br/upload/S/1983-2451/2011/v36n1/a1924.pdf>. Accessed on: 13 August 2017.

STANLEY, S. D.; KNYCH, H. D.; BLACK, J. B. Permitted medications: non-steroids anti-inflammatory medication. Available at: < http://ncha-sf-staging.azurewebsites.net/docs/default-source/default-document-library/medication_factsheet.pdf?sfvrsn=0 >. Accessed on: 26 August 2017.

STEEL, C. M.; PANNIRSELVAM, R. R.; ANDERSON, G. A. Risk of septic arthritis after intra-articular medication: a study of 16,624 injections in Thoroughbred racehorses. **Australian Veterinary Journal**, v. 91, n. 7, p. 268-273, 2013.

SUTTER, W. W.; BERTONE, A. L. Infections of muscle, joint, and bone. In: SELLON, D. C. S.; LONG, M. T. **Equine Infectious Diseases**. China: Elsevier, 2007. p. 62-66.

SVALA, E.; JIN, C.; RUETSCHI, U.; EKMAN, S.; LINDAHL, A.; KARLSSON, N. G.; SKIOLDEBRAND, E. Characterisation of lubricin in synovial fluid from horses with osteoarthritis. **Equine Veterinary Journal**, v. 49, n. 1, p. 116-123, 2015.

TARTANIUK, D. **Tarsal anatomy of the horse**. Available at: <https://www.slideshare.net/dvmfun/tarsal-anatomy-of-the-horse>. Accessed on: 12 January 2017.

THOMSEN, L. N.; THOMSEN, P. D.; DOWING, A.; TALBOT, R.; BERG, L. C. FOXO1, PXK, PYCARD and SAMD9L are differentially expressed by fibroblast-like cells in equine synovial membrane compared to joint capsule. **Biomedical Central Veterinary Research,** v. 13, n. 106, p. 01-08, 2017.

TODHUNTER, R. J. Anatomy and physiology of synovial joints. In: MCILWRAITH, C. W.; TROTER, G. W. **Joint disease in the horse**. Philadelphia: Saunders, 1996. p. 1-28.

VENDRUSCOLO, C. P. **Biomaterials and cell therapy in the repair of articular cartilage in horses**. 2011.19f. Final Coursework (Veterinary Medicine and Zootechnics) - State University of São Paulo (UNESP), Botucatu, 2011.

VIEIRA, F.A. **Diagnosis and treatment of septic arthritis in horses.** 2009. 37f Course completion work (Veterinary Medicine Course) - Faculdades Metropolitanas Unidas, São Paulo, 2009.

VOS, N. J.; DUCHARME, N. G. Analysis of factors influencing prognosis in foals with septic arthritis. **Irish Veterinary Journal**, v. 61, n. 2, p. 102-106, 2008.

WARREN, K. L. H.; WONG, D. M.; FULKERSON, C. V.; WANG, C.; SUN, Y. Bacterial isolates, antimicrobial susceptibility patterns, and factors associated with infection and outcome in foals with septic arthritis: 83 cases (1998-2013). **Journal of the American Veterinary Medicine Association**, v.246, n.7, p. 785-793, 2015.

WEEREN, P. R. V. General anatomy and physiology of joints. In: MCILWRAITH, C. W.; FRISBIE, D. D.; KAWCAK, C. E.; WEEREN, P. R.V. **Joint disease in the horse**. 2.ed. China: Elsevier, 2016, p. 1-20.

WEEREN, P. R. V. Septic Arthritis. In: MCILWRAITH, C. W.; FRISBIE, D. D.; KAWCAK, C. E.; WEEREN, P. R. V. **Joint Disease in the Horse.** 2.ed. China: Elsevier, 2016. p. 91-104.

WRIGHT, L.; EKSTROM, C. T.; KRISTOFFERSEN, M.; LINDEGAARD, C. Haematogenous septic arthritis in foals: short- and long- term outcome and analysis of factors affecting prognosis. **Equine Veterinary Education**, v. 29, n. 6, p.328-336, 2016.

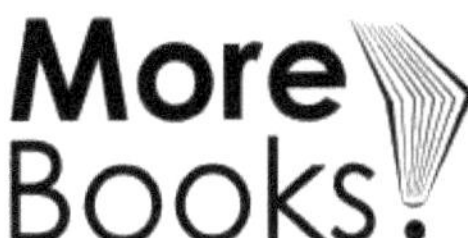

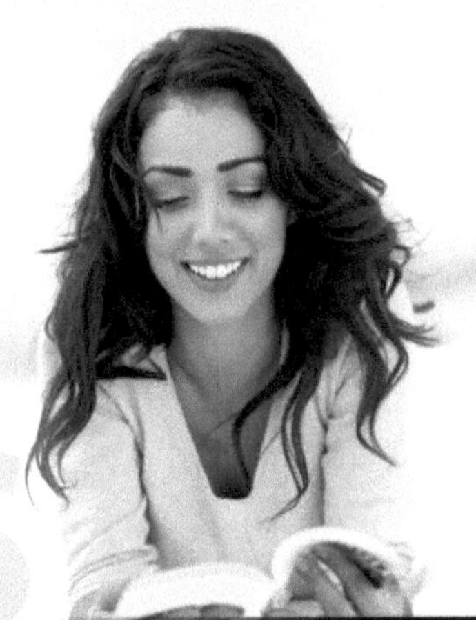

yes
I want morebooks!

Buy your books fast and straightforward online - at one of world's fastest growing online book stores! Environmentally sound due to Print-on-Demand technologies.

Buy your books online at
www.morebooks.shop

Kaufen Sie Ihre Bücher schnell und unkompliziert online – auf einer der am schnellsten wachsenden Buchhandelsplattformen weltweit! Dank Print-On-Demand umwelt- und ressourcenschonend produziert.

Bücher schneller online kaufen
www.morebooks.shop

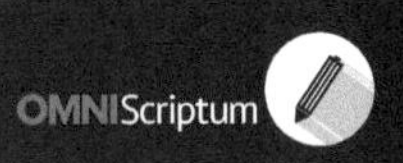

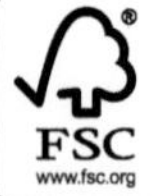

Printed by Books on Demand GmbH, Norderstedt / Germany